ASPERGERS SYNDROME

Get a More Extensive Learning About Asperger's

(A Complete Guide on Aspergers Symptoms)

Dona Matteson

Published by Tomas Edwards

© **Dona Matteson**

All Rights Reserved

Aspergers Syndrome: Get a More Extensive Learning About Asperger's (A Complete Guide on Aspergers Symptoms)

ISBN 978-1-990268-74-8

All rights reserved. No part of this guide may be reproduced in any form without permission in writing from the publisher except in the case of brief quotations embodied in critical articles or reviews.

Legal & Disclaimer

The information contained in this book is not designed to replace or take the place of any form of medicine or professional medical advice. The information in this book has been provided for educational and entertainment purposes only.

The information contained in this book has been compiled from sources deemed reliable, and it is accurate to the best of the Author's knowledge; however, the Author cannot guarantee its accuracy and validity and cannot be held liable for any errors or omissions. Changes are periodically made to this book. You must consult your doctor or get professional medical advice before using any of the suggested remedies, techniques, or information in this book.

Upon using the information contained in this book, you agree to hold harmless the Author from and against any damages, costs, and expenses, including any legal fees potentially resulting from the application of any of the information provided by this guide. This disclaimer applies to any damages or injury caused by the use and application, whether directly or indirectly, of any advice or information presented, whether for breach of contract, tort, negligence, personal injury, criminal intent, or under any other cause of action.

You agree to accept all risks of using the information presented inside this book. You need to consult a professional medical practitioner in order to ensure you are both able and healthy enough to participate in this program.

Table of Contents

INTRODUCTION 1

CHAPTER 1: WHAT IS ASPERGER SYNDROME? 4

CHAPTER 2: ASPERGER'S SYNDROME 18

CHAPTER 3: RAISING A CHILD WITH ASPERGER'S 38

CHAPTER 4: WHAT IS ASPERGER'S SYNDROME? 52

CHAPTER 5: WAYS THAT ADULTS CAN HELP A CHILD WITH AS UNDERSTAND WHAT IS SAID TO THEM 76

CHAPTER 6: THE IMPACT OF ASPERGER'S SYNDROME ACROSS THE LIFESPAN 86

CHAPTER 7: HELPING LOVED ONES COPE WITH ASPERGER'S SYNDROME 94

CHAPTER 8: MISUNDERSTANDINGS AND MISJUDGMENTS OF THE SOCIAL SURROUNDINGS 100

CONCLUSION 133

Introduction

Asperger's syndrome is a complex condition which belongs to autism spectrum disorder or (ASD). It is challenge that affects both children and adults. The child will experience challenges from this condition mainly in social interaction and more so nonverbal communication. The child will have repetitive and also restricted patterns of behavior and also interests. It belongs to the broad autism disorder group that inhibits normal productivity of the child. The person will have clumsy tendencies and a haltingly use of language. So this book will help you know how to handle this problem in children and even in adults and you will not be disadvantaged. In this book you will learn:

The indications of Asperger's Syndrome which range from modest to severe and may vary from one child to another. Children who suffer from this condition will experience a great challenge when it comes to socializing and interacting with their friends. At other times they will behave in an unconventional and awkward manner when it comes to social gathering. To make friendship for them is an arduous task. They will also face difficulties in beginning and sustaining a conversation. It is this challenge in their social skills that a lot of care and time have to be spent.

Asperger's syndrome is a condition that affects development and the social interaction of an individual. A full diagnosis cannot be fully realized until maximum and conclusive inputs have been put by several parties which include parents, teachers, doctors and caregivers who know the child or the adult very well after a time of observation. When these criteria are met, then one can full declare that the child or person is a victim of Asperger's Syndrome.

In summary, the criteria include unusual behavior, interests, social interaction and activities. The diagnosis will also include delay in language development, delay in self-help skills and curiosity in the child about the environment they live in.

I hope you will enjoy reading this book and be of help to the affected for it is teamwork that will help the people.

Chapter 1: What Is Asperger Syndrome?

Asperger Syndrome: An Overview

Asperger syndrome is a one of the five syndromes or development disorder in the autism spectrum. Asperger syndrome was first identified by the physician called Hans Asperger. He was observing the different behaviour traits in a group of students and he found that four boys with normal intelligence and cognition were exhibiting behaviours similar to an Autism child. In the year 1944, Hans Asperger published a paper in which he has described his observations of the Asperger syndrome and its various behaviour traits in children. Earlier people thought that the disorder is typically high functioning Autism. But then people understood that Asperger syndrome has many dissimilarities as compared to Autism. So he defined Asperger syndrome as a complex development disorder marked by impairments in communication, socialization, cognition, and sensation.

A person diagnosed with Asperger syndrome has many issues related to his behaviour and he faces many problems in socializing and communicating with other people. Asperger syndrome is different from the classic Autism and is considered as a neurological disorder that affects a person's ability to communicate and relate to others. It is a lifelong disorder and carries considerable and long-term behaviour problems.

Some Common Symptoms of Asperger Syndrome

The characteristics of Asperger syndrome differs from person to person, but the normal symptoms of this disorder are as follows: --

Troubles in understanding social behaviour and conversational language skills.

Hindrance to non functional routine or ritual.

Repetition of words and phrases.

Problems in normal functioning of fine motor skills and sensory integration.

A relevant preoccupation with objects or narrowly focused topics of interest.

Researches show that every 1 child out of 250 is diagnosed with Asperger syndrome in U.S. alone and this graph is a little bit higher in developing countries. Asperger syndrome is not easy to diagnose as its symptoms are not easy to recognize. Many common children show these symptoms during any phase in their life but a child suffering from Asperger syndrome has excess amount of the symptoms described above and that's why they face many obstacles in their day to day life.

Children suffering from Asperger syndrome have to face many conundrums during the initial phase of their life because they are not consciously aware that a certain disease is the main reason of their behaviour, functional, and cognition abilities. It is important to note in case of Asperger syndrome that these behaviour traits are neurologically based and do not include the individual's wilful understanding and disobedience. Asperger syndrome is one of the five Pervasive

Development Disorders that vary in different patients depending on their severity of symptoms, age, and presence of other mental disorders like mental retardation.

What Causes Asperger Syndrome?

Researchers are still doubtful about the real cause of Asperger syndrome. However, they have found that it tends to run in families suggesting that it may be hereditary and inherited from parent to child. Many researchers think that since Asperger is one of the Autistic disorders, so the root cause of this disease would be same as of Autism. Although, the precise causes of autism have not been identified but they found that a genetic component is involved in the main cause of autism. In some cases, autistic disorder may be the outcome of toxic exposure, problems during pregnancy, or prenatal infections. These environmental influences increase the chances of children suffering from autism or autism related dysfunctions like Asperger syndrome.

Impact of Asperger Syndrome on Children's Normal Life

How Asperger Syndrome Look Like?

As mentioned above, a child suffering from Asperger syndrome has many characteristics that involve impairment in socialization, cognition, communication, and sensation. These impairments are different among different children and exist on a continuum that varies from severity to minor impairment. As each individual suffering from Asperger syndrome is different, it sometimes become quite difficult to cope with them. The people who have to face these children often find it difficult to cope with the day to day changing behavioural features. It can often seem that the student you teach today is totally different person from the student you taught yesterday. On the basis of thorough research done by some specialists on Asperger syndrome, following are the common characteristics of persons with Asperger syndrome: --

Social Challenges

Lack of understanding of social cues.

Interpreting other children's word.

Difficulty engaging in reciprocal conversation.

Tendency to speak repeatedly without putting any impact on the listener.

Focus on the single topic of interest.

Communication Challenges

Difficulty in understanding some social nuances like sarcasm or metaphor.

Repeating last words without any proper meaning.

Poor judgement of personal space e.g. standing too close to other students.

Abnormal eye contact behaviour.

Unrelated facial expressions and gestures.

Cognition Challenges

Poor problem solving and organizational skills.

Obsessive and narrowly defined interests.

Concrete, literal thinking.

Problems in generalization and application of learned knowledge and skills across various situations, settings, and people.

Sensory and Motor Challenges

Over or under sensitivity to some sort of sensory stimuli like pain.

Difficulty in minor motor activities like writing.

Affect of Asperger Syndrome on a Child

Asperger syndrome has many social and behavioural issues that make a child lose control over his day to day life. As described earlier, in Asperger syndrome a child doesn't proactively behave in different manner than other children of his age but this behaviour is directly connected to the neurological disorders of his brain due to this disease. Following are some common issues that a child suffering from Asperger syndrome has to face in his day to day life: --

Socialization

Human being is a social animal and we cannot live alone in this world without any social exposure to us. Every child needs his social space to grow and develop into a complete human being. But a child suffering from Asperger syndrome deprives of the social exposure that he or she must need to grow into a perfect human being. Social impairments are the greatest challenges for students with this disorder. Every child needs a friend to develop his social skills in the society but Asperger syndrome deprives his natural instinct to make friends and he or she gets deflected from his peer students. Building and maintaining social friendships is very hard for a child suffering from this disease because of the student's lack of understanding of social issues, interpretation of other's words, and comprehension problems. This is the main reason why many students suffering from Asperger syndrome become a target of bullying, teasing, and victimization by their peers. Some common socialization problems of a child suffering from Asperger syndrome is described below: --

Conversational style: -- Individuals suffering from Asperger syndrome show lack of conversational skills and exhibit one sided interaction that may not be interested to his or her conversational partner or group. These individuals often get the impression of being talked at instead of participating in a reciprocal conversation. This lack of conversational skills is the main reason why these individuals are unable to communicate inside a social spectrum.

Signs of Bluntness: -- Children suffering from Asperger syndrome show signs of bluntness and often talk nonsense, which can make them look rude and insensitive. These children have a tendency to blurt out exactly what comes into mind without analysing whether this sentence is plausible in the situation or not.

Lack of implementing social rules: -- Students of Asperger syndrome lack the common skills of implementing any social rule to certain condition or circumstances. They learn social skills without fully understanding when and how to implement them. One of the common examples of this may be recurring burping. Burping is acceptable among young boys when they are with their peers. But recurring burping should be considered as an abnormal behaviour if you do it in the middle of your class's period. Most boys can understand this fact that recurring burping in public is neither polite nor an acceptable behaviour. But a child suffering from Asperger syndrome doesn't understand the changes in social setting and he should do repetitive burping in the middle of a class mistakenly perceiving burping to be socially acceptable.

Communication

Children suffering from Asperger syndrome generally have a good grammar and vocabulary skills that surpass their typically developing peers in some cases but they experience verbal and non-verbal communication deficits. Some common communication challenges that these children face is as follows: --

Social aspects of language: -- Children having Asperger syndrome are often found to behave in a somewhat different manner in case of language learning skills as compared to the peers of their age. These children often indulge themselves into detailed discussion of a single topic, which is of little or no interest to others. They also speak in exaggeration or in a monotone fashion, which seems weird between the age group of these children. They often shows a psychiatric disorder of language called 'Echolalia' which refers to the repetition of some else's spoken words with little or no social meaning. Children suffering from Asperger syndrome shows lack of common understanding of some famous English phrases like 'I heard it on the grapevine' or 'Elvis is out of building' these phrases have different meaning depending on the context they are used but a child suffering from Asperger syndrome would take the exact meaning of these sentences and 'I heard it on the grapevine' would make no sense in their terms of understanding the language.

Abstract concepts: -- Many languages need a precise understanding of abstract concepts like metaphors, parables, phrases, irony, sarcasm, and idioms. These concepts are the common building blocks of many languages and understanding them is mandatory for a child to learn the language properly. But children suffering from Asperger syndrome have to struggle a lot for learning languages having these concepts.

Body language and non-verbal communication: -- Children with Asperger syndrome find it difficult to behave normally in the social settings of their atmosphere with their body language and non-verbal communication. Some common examples of these deficits include limited or unrelated facial expressions and gestures, awkward body language, and social proximity i.e. standing to close or too far away in the social circle during a conversation. These children also face difficulty in understanding the facial expression and body language of other peers.

Cognition

Generally children suffering from Asperger syndrome have average and sometimes above average intelligence as compared to the peers of same age. They have a high concentration power and sometimes talk about topics way beyond their age level. However, Asperger syndrome is also responsible to create cognitive deficits that can lead to difficulties in academic activities. Some common examples of these deficits are as follows: --

Academic challenges: -- Despite having normal intelligence, children suffering from Asperger syndrome often experience cognitive difficulties that affect their academic achievements. These children found of having poor problem solving and organizational skills. They also lack concrete literal thinking and face difficulty to understand abstract concepts. These children become obsessive to a certain interest.

Emotions and stress: -- Asperger syndrome is a neurological disorder but the children suffering from it do not consciously choose to act like they often do and this is why when they are quite emotional rather logical in their decision making and behaviour. It is like as if the thinking centre of their brain becomes inactive while feeling centre started to act wildly. These children often seem to reactive without thinking in many cases.

Even if they learn more acceptable behaviours, they still act abnormal under stress and come to their default aggressive behaviour.

Inability to generalize knowledge: -- Asperger syndrome children have effective memorization skills but they store the information inside their mind as disconnected set of facts and despite having great memory, these children experience difficulty in applying information and use proper set of their knowledge.

Chapter 2: Asperger's Syndrome

What is Asperger's Syndrome?
This is a question that seems to be asked increasingly in our modern society. From engineers and computer programmers to quantum physicists, the highly intelligent but socially awkward populations of society are eventually beginning to find answers to the question they have always been busy with — "Why am I different?".

Tragically, the people who are asking the question are often people who should have been diagnosed with the condition earlier in life, but weren't, due to failures in the health and education systems. It is only now that famous celebrities are 'coming out' that Asperger's Syndrome is now in vogue.

According to medical sources, it is listed as a developmental disorder, but there is much more to it than that. It can be described as a 'hidden disability', meaning that you cannot recognise the condition from any outward appearance[1] (although the outside appearance can provide indicators).

It is important to note the manifestation of Asperger's Syndrome does vary from person to person. The below explanations are intended to be more of a guide than an absolute.

Later on in the book we will cover how Asperger's Syndrome has been incorporated into a wider diagnostic criteria of Autism. My personal opinion is that Asperger's Syndrome is deserving of its own category because we do have different lifestyles and capabilities.

Below is the official diagnosis criteria that was used in the Diagnostic and Statistical Manual, version four (DSM-IV).

"(I) Qualitative impairment in social interaction, as manifested by at least two of the following:

(A) marked impairments in the use of multiple nonverbal behaviors such as eye-to-eye gaze, facial expression, body posture, and gestures to regulate social interaction

(B) failure to develop peer relationships appropriate to developmental level

(C) a lack of spontaneous seeking to share enjoyment, interest or achievements with other people (e.g. by a lack of showing, bringing, or pointing out objects of interest to other people)

(D) lack of social or emotional reciprocity.

(II) Restricted repetitive & stereotyped patterns of behavior, interests and activities, as manifested by at least one of the following:

(A) encompassing preoccupation with one or more stereotyped and restricted patterns of interest that is abnormal either in intensity or focus

(B) apparently inflexible adherence to specific, nonfunctional routines or rituals

(C) stereotyped and repetitive motor mannerisms (e.g. hand or finger flapping or twisting, or complex whole-body movements)

(D) persistent preoccupation with parts of objects.

(III) The disturbance causes clinically significant impairments in social, occupational, or other important areas of functioning.

(IV) There is no clinically significant general delay in language (e.g. single words used by age 2 years, communicative phrases used by age 3 years).

(V) There is no clinically significant delay in cognitive development or in the development of age-appropriate self help skills, adaptive behavior (other than in social interaction) and curiosity about the environment in childhood.

(VI) Criteria are not met for another specific Pervasive Developmental Disorder or Schizophrenia."

Asperger's Syndrome (AS) has many behavioural signifiers, including difficulties in the three main areas of social communication, social interaction and social imagination. For example, subtleties in difference in tone of voice and facial expression, jokes, sarcasm, non-literal meanings and metaphors can be misunderstood, which often manifests as a perceptible social awkwardness. This can create difficulties in maintaining conventional friendships and relationships; behaviour may sometimes appear to others as clumsy or inappropriate due to an inability to read 'between the lines' and adhere to 'unwritten' social conventions. The most notable and dysfunctional characteristic of Asperger's is a lack of demonstrative empathy, which brings with it a lack of emotional and social reciprocity.[5] This, in turn, can often lead to other problems, such as feelings of isolation or depression or a strong belief within an individual that they somehow don't 'fit in'.

Another characteristic often associated with Asperger's is a difficulty to imagine more than one possible future outcome to set events; also there's a tendency to repeat a set pattern or patterns of behaviour, leading to a narrow or limited pursuit of rigid interests, such as an interest in numbers or specific details[1]. In children, this characteristic can manifest as a difficulty to engage in "let's pretend" games, and a preference instead for games involving logic or systems; for example a child with Asperger's may avoid the dressing up box but excel at maths or logic problems.

Technically, Asperger's Syndrome is classified as a type of Autism Spectrum Disorder, but for readers of this blog and our email course you will understand that there is some debate about how similar it actually is to Autism. People with the syndrome are often highly functioning and are able to cope and succeed in the world, unlike other people on the Autism Spectrum.

Recent medical studies have actually discovered that the brains of those with Asperger's Syndrome are different to those with classic Autism. You will also be interested to know that the exact symptoms develop differently in those with Asperger's. As far as classic Autism goes, many symptoms can be identified early but with Asperger's the symptoms come around a lot later.

The brains of people with Asperger's are fundamentally wired differently. Instead of thinking in language, like most people do, one is more likely to think in pictures if one has the syndrome.

In reality, what this means is an entirely different way of thinking about the world around them, producing extremely intelligent people who, in layman's terms, can do some of the most complicated tasks and find solutions to difficult problems.

The downside, of course, is that dealing with social situations becomes very difficult. When one thinks differently to the norm, it is very difficult to identify and communicate with others. Things that most people take for granted in the communication process, such as small talk and being able to identify the body language and emotions of other people, are often challenging. All of these skills are things that we believe can be learned, but the default position makes it very difficult.

Doctors are reluctant to make an official diagnosis due to miseducation or a preference to try and identify (and therefore treat) just the most prominent symptoms. We get many emails from people who are frustrated that their doctors won't recognise their condition.

[1] The Autism Society's website: http://www.autism.org.uk/about-autism/autism-and-asperger-syndrome-an-introduction/what-is-asperger-syndrome.aspx.

[2] Peer reviewed website kidshealth.org http://kidshealth.org/parent/medical/brain/asperger.html.

[3] Klin A. (2006). "Autism and Asperger syndrome: an overview". Rev. Bras. Psiquiatr. **28**(suppl. 1):S3–S11. doi:10.1590/S1516-44462006000500002. PMID 16791390.

[4] Baskin J.H., Sperber M., Price B.H. (2006). "Asperger syndrome revisited". Rev. Neurol. Dis. **3**(1):1–7.

[5] McPartland J., Klin A. (2006). "Asperger's syndrome". Adolesc. Med. Clin. **17**(3):771–788. doi:10.1016/j.admecli.2006.06.010. PMID 17030291.

Symptoms of Asperger's

Before we go into detail about the testing process for Asperger's we want to describe the symptoms that one may recognise. While the symptoms of Asperger's Syndrome do vary from person to person, you may identify with any of the following:

Inflexibility/attachment to routines

Someone with Asperger's usually prefers routines and can experience emotional upset if routines are altered.

The process of moving home or even going away for a weekend or a holiday can cause distress, as can a change of job or loss of a relationship.

It can also manifest in situations where the person is focused on a particular task and gets resentful when someone interrupts to make conversation or ask a question.

Difficulty engaging in conversation

Often people with Asperger's can have difficulty engaging in conversation as well as keeping eye contact with the person they are talking to. The conversation revolves around talking about a subject the person with AS is extremely interested in, while at the same time being unable to correctly interpret the social expressions of the person being spoken to. This often results in a failure to recognise whether the other person is interested in the topic and can lead to the person being spoken to becoming bored out of their brain. However, as social etiquette dictates that they not show it, this invariably sets up a vicious cycle, because unless the person with AS gets some concrete indication that the person is not interested, he will assume they are, and keep going.

The long-term outcome of this process is that people can tend to avoid the person with AS due to their lack of social skills.

Emotional awareness and responses

It is often said the people with AS have no emotional empathy, but I would suggest that this is a myth. In actual fact people with AS have a very strong emotional sensitivity for others.

It is true that it is often difficult for people with AS to respond to the emotions of others in the ways neurotypical (NT) people have come to expect, but it is not for lack of sensitivity.

I believe this, in part, comes from the difficulty in processing the emotions and sensory overload that occurs as a result of exposure to others' emotions. Very often this can result in withdrawal from the other person's emotions when the individual is unable to deal with both the feelings of the other and the feelings that they are also experiencing.

This has led to the belief that people with AS are cold and not empathetic.

Repetitive rituals and behaviours (stimming)

This can express itself in the engagement of repetitive rituals, such as body movements, habits and behaviours. Examples of this include hand flapping, twirling, rocking or obscure methods of play.

Stimming is usually a result of some form of anxiety or sensory overload where the person uses such motions to self sooth and feel better. It is one of the many misunderstood aspects of Autism and Asperger's. Many times children are prevented from stimming because it is deemed out of place but often, if left to stim, children will eventually release the anxiety that is causing the stimming and stop in a more calm space. If forcibly stopped, the anxiety continues only to potentially be expressed in another form, such as the (much less socially tolerated) meltdown, or through another, later, set of stims.

Sensory sensitivity

We will cover sensory issues in more detail later in the book, but we will also list it here to give you an idea what it is.

Sensory sensitivity occurs when a person has difficulty integrating and processing the various signals that enter the body through the senses. While this is often related to sound, it can also occur with the colour, texture, smell or taste of food; or it can result in a low tolerance of noises of certain frequencies.

Impaired motor skills

Sometimes one can experience an impairment of motor skills, such as those used in playing catch, riding a bike or tying shoelaces. Although not exclusive to AS, this can often be an effect of the disorder.

From the outside, this looks like clumsiness or laziness, but in fact it is a condition and side effect, which makes hand–eye coordination and balance very difficult. There is also an anxiety associated with this aspect of AS, due to an apprehension of being required to perform some motor-based activity.

Special interests

Those with AS tend to develop special interests. A special interest is a particular hobby or subject that the person tends to become obsessed with. Often the person knows the subject inside out and develops an intense passion for it.

I believe this is one of the reasons adults with AS often excel at areas of science, engineering and computing. A high focus on one particular area makes the person an expert in the field. The downside of this, however, is that the person will have difficulty in stepping back and taking time away from their special interest.

Repetitive behaviours

This can include odd behaviours, such as lining up objects in a row or obsessively talking about the same subject repeatedly. Obsessions about eating (which foods to eat first, which foods should/should not be combined, etc.); methods of playing and/or certain routines are also strong indicators of this condition.

Autism vs Asperger's Syndrome

Sometimes within this book and on the Asperger's Test Site we use the words 'Autism' and 'Asperger's' interchangeably. While there is a lot of debate still as to whether Asperger's and Autism are the same, we thought that it was good to explain more at this point.

Leo Kanner was the first person to describe the nature of Autism and its symptoms almost sixty years ago. Later, Hans Asperger wrote about a condition, which was first termed 'autistic psychopathology' and is now known as Asperger's Syndrome. Though there were similarities in the two discoveries,

Asperger claimed that his disorder was not a variation of the initial Autism discovery.

According to the most widely used diagnostic tool, DSM-IV-TR (Diagnostic and Statistical Manual of Mental Disorders), both disorders are classified as Pervasive Developmental Disorders. Since 1994 Asperger's Syndrome was added to the fourth edition as a separate disorder.

Today the debate continues among academic researchers but there is a growing general consensus that Autism and Asperger's Syndrome are, in fact, two independent conditions, although Asperger's Syndrome had been incorporated under the umbrella of Autism to overcome clinical confusion between the diagnoses of these syndromes.

These differences are based on the different language and cognitive challenges that those with Autism and AS face.

Communication differences

Individuals with more severe forms of autism are more likely to show symptoms of limited communication skills, both verbal and non-verbal.

Diagnostic differences

Autism can be detected early, usually at the age of five, while those with AS often remain undiagnosed until eleven years old. The late onset of complex problems with social skills explains how and why people with AS are diagnosed later than their counterparts with Autism.

Studies conducted at Monash University conclude that children with Autism portray a particular style of walking; this will be fundamental in the early diagnosis of Autism as children learn to walk before they develop social skills.

Social, motor & cognitive differences

Children with Autism have limited interest in events, items and the people in their environment. They tend to favour repeated actions. Children with AS are less likely to show delays in age-appropriate skills, such as self-help, curiosity and the ability to adapt.

Autistic children, in many instances, are characterised by having motor difficulties and tend to be preoccupied with parts of objects such as the wheels of a toy car; their limited and circumscribed interest consumes a great deal of their time. Individuals with AS are less likely to display these symptoms.

Children with Autism usually have cognitive delays from early infancy. Children with AS do not tend to show this kind of delay; they might be quite talented in numeric abilities, learning to read, and being constructive in memory games.

Similarities in social & behavioural skills

Autism and High-functioning Autism (HFA) have several common characteristics with Asperger's Syndrome (AS). AS and HFA individuals have normal cognitive abilities and do not experience any significant delay in acquiring language skills.

Individuals with Autism and Asperger's Syndrome are similar in terms of their inability to create and maintain social relationships. The verbal expression of an individual with Autism might be limited or even non-existent, although certain characteristics can also be observed in individuals with Asperger's Syndrome. Despite their developed vocabulary and normal intelligence, they are unable to socialise in an acceptable manner. Their speech is overly formal and/or too literal. During interactions with peers their behaviour is deemed socially and emotionally inappropriate; this is also true for individuals with Autism. They possess similar traits in their inability to understand non-verbal signs and gestures.

Both individuals with Autism and Asperger's Syndrome have a similar behavioural profile; hence the same treatment methods can be affective for both groups. This is why some clinicians and researchers suggest that it is inappropriate to talk about two separate conditions or different disorders. A dimensional, rather than a categorical, view of Autism and Asperger's Syndrome seems to be more reasonable.

Differences in degrees of sociability

Delays and disturbances of communication are more explicit in Autism. Individuals with Asperger's Syndrome might be able to successfully complete school or find a job, which is unlikely for individuals with Autism. People with AS will experience significant impairment in important areas of functioning; for example, social interactions or correct occupational behaviour.

Important factors in their differences

The main worry in defining Asperger's Syndrome as a lesser form of Autism is that it could imply that children with AS do not face as many difficulties as those with Autism, whereas, in fact, they can suffer far more severe anxiety disorders and depression than those with Autism.

Another important factor is that the parents of those diagnosed with Asperger's Syndrome are able to be given guidelines to assist their children to develop fulfilling social activities and a chance to explore successful career options.

Further studies

Due to deeper understanding of these disorders, such as the brain cell suppression in HFA, which is not present in those with AS, resulting in variants in diagnostic tests and subsequent treatments, sufferers of both syndromes can be diagnosed and treated with the most appropriate methods. With ongoing studies into the psychological and brain differences between these syndromes, it will aid the future development of diagnostic tools and subsequent treatments for each disorder.

Chapter 3: Raising A Child With Asperger's

Development of Social Communication in Children with Asperger's Syndrome:

Communication does not merely include the ability to use words, but includes body language, facial expression, and tone of voice. These non-verbal cues often reveal what people think or feel when they are using particular words. For example, the same word spoken with different gestures represents a different concept. To be successful communicators, we have to know how to interpret and respond to these cues, and how to use them ourselves.

In childhood, most of the infants start noticing non-verbal cues by observing their parents using facial expressions to support, acknowledge, scold, or scare them. On the other hand, children with Asperger's have difficulty in 'tuning in' to the context of the words, feelings, and thoughts of others. This ability does not develop at the same pace as in other children.

It is difficult for them to empathize, and to have insight into what others are thinking. As they do not know how to behave in social situations, such children may find it hard to make friends and to build relationships with other people.

Fortunately, children with Asperger's Syndrome can experience an improvement in developing their social communication skills. Research has shown that if extra help and support from family members is given, children with Asperger's can learn many vital skills that can help them connect and make friendships with others.

The Hanen Centre commits to supporting adults who live with individuals with Asperger's Syndrome, including parents, caregivers, early childhood educators, and speech-language pathologists. The Centre provides them with the knowledge and tools they need to promote social communication skills.

Key to social interaction is to take others' perspectives: The children who are most successful in making friends are those who can see and understand the points of view of others.

Parents and caregivers play an essential role: In a child's life, family plays the most important role, and parents should know how to intervene for their children.

Learning happens naturally: It is while children are having everyday conversations and activities with their parents and other family members that they can learn to communicate the best.

Many of the treatments that are carried out for Asperger's Syndrome are based on teaching patients a script that they need to follow in social situations. The Hanen Center has developed a program called 'Talk Ability' to empower parents to help their child develop the social skills needed to make them a successful communicator.

Talk Ability Program for Parents:

The research conducted in the Talk Ability Program shows that the children who converse with others about their thoughts and feelings start to attune themselves to the thoughts of others. This is also called the Theory of Mind, the knowledge and awareness that other people have their own private thoughts. This fact is used to create child's ability to have successful relationships.

Studies have shown that when words such as Think, Remember, or Wonder are used by parents in conversations with children, the children learn these words and start to talk in the same way. When parents use the correct vocabulary, children start talking and thinking differently. They know how important it is to listen and understand ideas and the perspectives of others. In this way, parents can significantly improve overall social and communication skills.

With an integrated approach of Hanen, parents get the benefits of learning how to make the best of their child's interests, preferences, and daily routine to naturally improve communication skills. Parents and therapists work together to deepen and increase learning opportunities for the child.

Asperger's is on the milder end of PDD. Kids with Asperger's usually have normal intelligence and normal language acquisition at early stages, though it is difficult for them to interact socially and communicate non-verbally. They may also show persevering or recurring behaviors.

Preschool: A preschool-aged Asperger's child may have difficulty understanding the basics of social interaction. They may have difficulty picking up on social cues, and have the desire to make friends but be unable to.

Elementary School: Children with Asperger's cannot use the appropriate volume or tone for their speech, an issue known as "poor pragmatic language skills." They may be standing too close or unable to make eye contact while speaking. It may not be possible for them to understand humor, metaphors, or slang expressions. As compared to other children, kids with Asperger's may become highly obsessed with some topics. Change has to be gradual or sometimes even unnoticeable to not be hugely disruptive to their lives.

Middle and High School: The most difficult time is during middle and high school. Milder forms of Asperger's may be diagnosed and given treatment at this level, since they might have been unnoticeable before this age. Social demands may become more complex during adolescence. An increase in opposition or aggressive behavior may be shown.

Adulthood: Some people with Asperger's Syndrome may have learned to compensate enough to make them indistinguishable from a non-Asperger's person. They can carry out everyday routines and go through life normally, getting married, holding jobs, and having kids. They may be able to do technical jobs very well, but when it comes to being social, their job may become more challenging. Some can do well with predictable cyclic work, while others enjoy facing complex technical problem-solving.

Associated Difficulties: People with Asperger's may have difficulty learning, and may possess a short attention span. In fact, individuals may first be diagnosed with ADHD rather than Asperger's Syndrome. Children with ADHD can also have social difficulties, but the main difference between the two conditions is that ADHD individuals are not able to concentrate, and are hyperactive and impulsive. They find themselves very different from others, which may lead them to depression that may continue if not treated.

Involvement of Parents: Parents play a vital role in developing behavior patterns in children. Children with Asperger's need extra attention and time. A parent must learn to differentiate between the willful disobedience of a child and a misunderstanding about social cues. Try to reduce the tension when you sense that the child is being overloaded emotionally. Parents should prepare other family members to change their routine according to the child's needs. The babysitter for such children should be chosen carefully, and play dates should be appropriately managed by parents since Asperger's children are often happier with similar kids. Parents can help teachers understand the unique behavior of their child. Parenting any adolescent can be a difficult task, but teens with Asperger's are often socially disengaged at this stage, so they may not be ready for the same kind of freedom as others. If you can find another child with Asperger's who is slightly older then the age of your own child, they can act as a guide to help them understand how to dress, or use certain slang. If that mentor is going to the same school, they can be a guide there as well.

Adults may get an advantage from group therapy or individual behavioral therapy. Some therapists can work on adults for pragmatic language skills. A person with Asperger's can be helped by behavioral coaching. For associated problems such as depression and anxiety, drugs may be needed, but it is important to understand the individual's condition because some people do not need medication. They can get a suitable job that relies on their strengths, focus on having small social circles, and become productive members of society.

Helping a Child with Asperger's:

Providing the child with support and love within the home environment is important. Remember that a child with Asperger's is just like other children, with their own strengths, weaknesses, and needs. Give them unconditional support, and try to understand them as much as you can.

Educate yourself about the condition so that you know what to expect, which is very important for helping the child develop independence and success in and out of the house. Following are a few suggested points on how to help a child with Asperger's Syndrome better integrate into society and learn to manage their symptoms. If you can be flexible, creative, and willing to learn more about your child, this will help you raise a child to be happy, healthy member of their family and of society.

General strategies for success:

Children with Asperger's syndrome get advantages from daily routines for meals, homework, and bedtime. They also like precise rules and schedules, which mean less stress and uncertainty for them.

Many people do best with spoken (rather than nonverbal) instructions and homework. A direct, brief, and clear-cut method may also be helpful.

People with Asperger's often have difficulty understanding the "big picture" and are likely to see only part of a situation rather than the whole. This is why they frequently benefit from a "parts-to-whole" teaching approach.

Image supports, which may include graphic schedules and other printed materials that serve as managerial aids, can be helpful.

Be alert that background noises that may seem minor or unnoticeable to you, such as a clock ticking or the hum of fluorescent lighting, can disturb your child.

Children with Asperger's may be particularly interested in video games, computers, or other screen-based media such as TV. If possible, keep televisions, video games, and computers out of your child's bedroom. When children with Asperger's have these devices in their bedroom, they are more likely to sleep fewer hours, especially for video games. If your child doesn't get enough sleep, their symptoms may be worse.

Children often mature more slowly as a result of Asperger's. Don't always expect them to "act their age."

Try to spot stress triggers and evade them if possible. Prepare your child in advance of new or tricky situations, and teach them ways to take care of themselves. For example, teach your child coping skills for dealing with a change or new situations.

Strategies for developing social skills:

It is difficult for children with Asperger's to understand the rules of a society that come naturally to other children. It is your responsibility to inform them about why a particular behavior and response is required in certain situations.

Support your child in finding out how to communicate with other people, how to respond when others ask questions, and why this response is important. Praise them for their efforts, particularly when they use their communication skills without prompting.

Games, question-and-answer sessions, and other practice activities should be held by family members. These activities may call for taking turns or putting yourself in other's place.

By role-playing and pointing out human behavior in movies, you can help your child recognize the feelings of people around them. Tell them about how you are feeling and your reactions, and become a role model for them.

Educate your child about reading and responding accurately to social cues. Teach them how to use rote phrases in various situations, such as asking for an apology or when being introduced. By role playing, help your child understand how to interact.

Foster involvement of other family members if the child tends to be a loner.

Educate your child about what is appropriate in public or private places. Hugging people they've just met is not suitable in public, but is fine in private.

Strategies for school:

Visual systems such as calendars, checklists and notes can be used by teachers to classify and arrange the school work.

Walk through the child's schedule before their school years start. Pictures can also be used to orient your child to the new settings and environment before they start going o school.

Bullying and teasing by other children should be eliminated by keeping a strict eye on all students. You should talk to the child's teacher or a counselor about educating classmates about Asperger's Syndrome.

Ask the teacher to place your child next to classmates who are more responsive to your child's particular needs. These classmates can also become buddies during a recess period or at lunch.

Your child should be encouraged by teachers to take part in class activities that focus their academic skills, such as vocabulary, reading, and art.

Set a specific time for homework and make it a habit of to do assignments at certain time. This way your child will learn how to manage their time.

To motivation a child, rewards can be given. Let them watch TV or play their favorite video game. You can also give them points towards his special interests when you think he is performing well.

Many children have naturally poor handwriting. To make homework easier, typing on a computer can be helpful, and can also improve motor skills and informational organization. Occupational therapy can also help significantly in some cases.

Chapter 4: What Is Asperger's Syndrome?

Asperger's syndrome is a developmental disorder related to the autistic spectrum but at a much higher level of functioning. Unlike those with autism, those who have Asperger's syndrome generally learn the same way average people do, learning to speak at a young age and eventually attending school in the same classes and at the same age of their peers. Like autism, however, those with Asperger's syndrome may have trouble understanding social or communication skills. This often results in being viewed as 'weird' by those around them who aren't familiar with the disorder.

Asperger's syndrome is typically diagnosed at an early age, but because those who have it are on the higher functioning end of the autism scale, it can go undiagnosed well into adulthood. This has been especially common in the past when the disorder wasn't as well known and understood as it has become in recent years. Similar to autism, there is no cure and the exact cause of the disorder is unknown, however, it is possible to manage the symptoms, including clumsiness, obsessive routines, and sensitivity to environmental changes. This is done with behavioral therapy, resulting in many adults with Asperger's syndrome appearing mostly 'normal' with the exception of lack of social skills.

The lack of social skills doesn't mean that all adults with Asperger's appear rude, but rather they have trouble understanding social cues. For example, it's not uncommon for those with Asperger's syndrome to share a deep passion for something, whether it be horses or molecules. They may want to talk about this passion constantly, despite the listener growing visibly annoyed. This is because they don't understand that sighing or looking at a watch means the listener is uninterested.

Due to this extreme passion, many adults with Asperger's syndrome end up excelling in careers involving their interest. It's not uncommon for adults with Asperger's to become CEO's or other high ranking positions because unlike other employees, they don't spend their time socializing with others, but rather learning as much as humanly possible about their passion.

What is the Asperger Syndrome diagnostic scale?

The Asperger Syndrome Diagnostic Scale, also known as ASDS, is a tool used to screen for children who might meet criteria for Asperger's Syndrome. This quickly administered standardized test only takes approximately 15 minutes to complete. It is appropriate for children ages five through 18 years old.

The screening tool is standardized and uses percentiles to give an AS Quotient. This score predicts the likelihood that a child or adolescent has Asperger's Syndrome. The test covers behaviors across several domains, including cognitive, maladaptive, social, sensory, motor, and language.

The behaviors addressed are those behaviors typically seen in children with Asperger's, as well as behaviors that are seen in children without an Autistic Disorder.

The Asperger Syndrome Diagnostic Scale has an administrative qualification level of B. This means that individuals who administer the ASDS must have a degree from an accredited four-year college. This degree must be completed in psychology, counseling, or speech and language pathology. The individual must also have completed coursework in test interpretation, psychometrics, educational statistics, or measurement theory or a license indicating appropriate training in the ethics and competency required for using psychological tests.

The respondent for the ASDS can be one of several individuals who are very familiar with the child or adolescent being tested. Parents and siblings are often the primary respondents.

The child's service providers, such as speech and language pathologists, therapists, and teachers can also act as respondents.

The Asperger Syndrome Diagnostic Scale cannot be used in isolation to provide a diagnosis of Asperger's. The ASDS is a screening tool to indicate the likelihood of the individual having Asperger's. The AS Quotient can be used to indicate whether a professional should further evaluate the child in order to receive an official formal diagnosis.

One concern with the ASDS is that it has not been shown to reliably differentiate between Asperger Syndrome and the other subtypes of Autism Spectrum Disorder. Since the symptoms of Asperger are also similar to the symptoms of PDD-NOS and Autistic Disorder, a qualified team of autism professionals must do further evaluation. This can help determine what subset of Autism Spectrum Disorder the individual has.

A benefit of the ASDS is that it not only provides an overall AS Quotient, but it also gives scores for each of the individual domains on the test. The individual results in the cognitive, language, social, maladaptive, and sensor motor subscales can assist the professional in determining specific areas of deficit and difficulty in the child. These scores can be especially helpful in treatment planning and determining areas for further testing.

The results of the ADSD also have other non-clinical purposes. They can also be used to help draft goals for the child's IEP or school intervention plan. The test can also be given annually as a way to measure growth and progress across the different domains in an individual already diagnosed with Asperger Syndrome.

What types of Asperger's tests are available for adults?

Like previously stated, Asperger syndrome is a pervasive developmental disorder characterized by significant impairments in social interaction and stereotyped patterns of behavior. What distinguishes Asperger Syndrome from other Autism Spectrum Disorders is the lack of any significant delay in language or cognitive ability. Asperger Syndrome is not as easy to diagnose as other disorders of the Autism Spectrum, so it is quite common for a person with Asperger to receive the diagnosis as an adult, even though the problems began in childhood. There are several tests and assessments that are designed to determine whether an adult has Asperger Syndrome or one of the other Autism Spectrum Disorders.

The ADI (Autism Diagnostic Interview-Revised) is an interview-based assessment that is used to ask questions of a parent, or if the parent is not available, some other person who knew the individual as a child. The questions are designed to determine whether the adult had problems with social interactions as a child and to rule out other forms of autism. The ADI is effective, but it is limited since the parent may no longer be available, and it takes about three hours to administer.

The AQ (Autism Spectrum Quotient) is a much shorter screening device used to identify adults who may have Asperger

Syndrome or Autism. This instrument contains 50 questions that relate to the areas of social skill, attention switching, attention to detail, communication and imagination. The subject responds to each question with "definitely agree," "slightly agree," "slightly disagree" and "definitely disagree." The responses to these questions show the degree to which the subject has features typical of people with Autism or Asperger Syndrome.

Another Asperger screening instrument is the EQ (Empathy Quotient), a 15 item questionnaire used to determine the degree to which an individual cannot understand the feelings and thoughts of others. Though this is a really short assessment that focuses on only one area of development, it has a very strong correlation with the presence of Asperger Syndrome.

Where does Asperger's come from?

So where does Asperger's comes from? Before I tell you, allow me to describe a quality which underlies the whole of Emergence Personality Theory. This quality? Blamelessness; the idea that no one consciously causes their pain. This includes the parents of kids with Asperger's. Not one of them ever causes their child to get Asperger's.

Where does it come from then? It was once normal for all of us to focus on sensation at the expense of our social relationships. When? In the first six months of life. Unfortunately, some babies never expand beyond this focus. Thus, they incur the condition we call, Kanner's Autism. In the second six months of life, we all have another norm. We focus on learning how to use the ability we mastered in our first six months; sensation itself, to sense the things in our environment. Here again, some few babies unfortunately never focus beyond this point. In their case, we call what they have, OCPD; Obsessive Compulsive Personality Disorder. The compulsion to sense the things in their environment at the expense of connecting to people.

And Asperger's then? Asperger's comes into being sometime during a baby's second year of life. How? Well, consider what is normal for babies to focus on during this stage in their lives. They focus on learning to understand the things they've learned to sense in the prior stage of their development. Thus, if babies do not move past this focus, they remain intensely interested in learning for learning's sake, even to the point wherein they never learn to connect to people.

Is there a fourth norm then? Absolutely. From age two to age four, kids normally rebel against any pressure put on them to simply parrot what other folks have learned. The "terrible two's," remember? So what does this turn out to be if the baby never loses this focus? ADD. Attention Deficit Disorder. And yes, I know medically minded folks now call this condition, ADHD. However, it seems incredibly silly to diagnose a kid as having ADHD without HD. Which happens to be the most common version of this lab rat label.

What could we be doing to better help these folks?

So what could we be doing to better help these folks? Well, in the case of Asperger's, we could be focusing our efforts on getting these folks to make "connecting" more important than "information." Note, I haven't simply said, teach them better social skills.

In truth, teaching mouth readers to read eyes is a lot easier than you might imagine. In fact, given they believe you have something valid to say, folks with Asperger's are among the best folks of all to teach.

What else could we be doing? We could stop telling them they have a disease. They do not. They have a style of relating to the world which was once normal for all of us but no longer is.

During this time, we all made learning the meaning of things our special interest. Moreover, in babies aged one to two, this focus is absolutely normal. In people with Asperger's, however, this tendency never leaves them. Thus, what was once normal now impairs their very ability to see the beauty in people. And renders them unable to do much more than parrot authentic social connections. The very thing that ADD kids hate doing. Which in part explains why AS kids have the most difficult time with ADD kids.

What else could we be doing to help? For one thing, we could pay more attention to the way "focusing on information more than people" plays out in the very nature of peoples' language skills.

"Fuzzy" and "fussy." Two very different qualities. Especially when applied to language. The ability to help here would come from teaching both those with Asperger's and those who do not have it, to speak to each other in the other's language. In effect, they both become bilingual, in that they both learn to speak "fussy" and they both learn to speak "fussy." Learning this alone has changed the whole outlook on the world.

As well as allowing them to socially connect to others for the first time in their life.

One more thing we could be doing is we could stop reminding people with

Asperger's that some few folks with Asperger's became world changers. Why stop saying this? Because this only makes them feel even more inept. And more like failures.

People with Asperger's are not failures. They are simply in the minority, both language wise and interest wise. Moreover, to see this as true, simply imagine our world were it not for people like them. Easier in some ways. Yes. Certainly. But without the special interests of those few who have changed the world?

HOW TO IDENTIFY ATYPICAL ASPERGERS SYNDROME?

The incidence of Asperger's Syndrome is on the rise. Asperger's is one of the Autistic Spectrum Disorders, or ASD's. Whenever we see a spike in the incidence of a disorder, I always ask the questions "is this disorder/syndrome occurring more frequently? Or, are we simply diagnosing it more often? Is it the new 'fashionable' diagnosis?" These are important professional questions. Labels and diagnoses can shape a future for the better or worse. We shouldn't diagnose lightly. Many implications follow a diagnosis.

I am seeing with more frequency, elements of Asperger's Syndrome in children but an absence of some key identifying symptoms. The diagnostic criteria listed in the Diagnostic and Statistical Manual IV (DSM-IV, the manual authorized by the American Psychiatric Association) is far too long to reprint here in a book. Some highlights are as follows:

1. Qualitative impairment in social interaction.

2. Restricted repetitive and stereotyped patterns of behavior, interests, and activities.

3. The disturbance causes clinically significant impairment in social, occupational, or other important areas of functioning.

4. There is no significant general delay in language (e.g., single words used by age 2 years, communicative phrases used by age 3 years).

5. There is no clinically significant delay in the cognitive development of age-appropriate self-help skills, adaptive behavior (other than in social interaction), and curiosity about the environment in childhood.

6. Criteria are not met for another specific Pervasive Developmental Disorder or Schizophrenia.

I am using the term in this chapter "Atypical Asperger's Syndrome" to refer to children who seem to meet some of the criteria but not all. Things just don't seem to click for these kids. They just don't engage the way other children do.

Atypical Aspergers may be best discussed by comparing it to some other possible diagnoses that we may be ruled out. They are as follows:

1. Social Anxiety Disorder: Children with this disorder may appear quite shy. They are hesitant to engage with other children. They prefer the company of adults. In differentiating this from Atypical Asperger's, the Asperger's child isn't remotely upset, concerned or bothered by

the fact that they aren't included in the group. Or, they are included in the group but remain somewhat permanently distant. They can play side by side with other children without really interacting with the other child.

2. Low Intellectual Functioning: Upon initial observation, the Atypical Aspergers child may appear dull or lacking in intelligence. The low intellectual functioning child generally will perform poorly in school and require basic skills level classes.

The Atypical Asperger's child, however, is most often bright. They do well on test despite appearing lost or disinterested.

Asperger's Syndrome children typically make poor eye contact, speak in limited phrases, are tangential, prefer social isolation. They display a lack of spontaneous seeking to share enjoyment, interests or achievements with others. They also display a lack of social or emotional reciprocity.

I am seeing Atypical Asperger's children who make good eye contact. They are often capable of conducting a conversation. Parents and teachers report that these children are less skilled in conversation with their peer age group. They may spontaneously share experiences or achievements but often at inappropriate times, interjecting such as a discussion somewhat randomly. And although they are bright, if I were their age I wouldn't be very interested in what they talk about. They appear immature because they are socially immature.

For some reason, the Atypical Asperger's child doesn't seem interested in athletics and also not very good at them. I don't fully understand the neurology involved but I'm suspecting a connection.

Fashionable Syndrome?

I was discussing Asperger's with my friend just last week. We were looking at the homes of America's richest tech guys, Bill Gates, Steve Jobs and "the facebook guy" Mark Zuckerberg. Our conversation led us to "how many of these very bright and creative guys have Asperger's." And we must make an important point, just because someone appears socially awkward doesn't mean that they have any disorder at all, let alone Aspergers. It was simply a conversation. I am not diagnosing any of these individuals from afar and have no idea if any of them have any version of Asperger's Syndrome. The point though is that he told me that in his 20 something age group it has become "fashionable" to say that you have Asperger's.

It is sort of a badge of honor and an easy explanation for ones "quirkiness" now in social situations. Guys in bars and clubs are using this to create an aura of "intellectual elite" associated with themselves. I see it as a way of saying "I'm really better and smarter than you and you couldn't possibly really understand me so don't even try." It's the new "I'm a nerd" declaration. Remember when being called a nerd was an insult? Remember when it became a badge of honor years later? This also points out that the more evident cases of adult Atypical Asperger's Syndrome occur in bright creative people.

I don't believe that the incidence is higher in bright people than less bright people. We simply notice it more because we notice high achievers overall more than lesser achievers.

This may seem strange or unusual at first glance. But think of how often you hear people referring to "my ADD." I hear this all the time. It's become an excuse for everything. Any time someone forgets fails to complete a project or return a phone call promptly, they announce that it's there ADD.

So to think that now the fashionable disorder or "disorder du jour" is something called Asperger's doesn't surprise me in the least.

We, as a society, are influenced by media and current fashion. All of the Autistic Spectrum disorders are in "fashion" in the media.

And this points to concern. Certain diagnoses become popular. Think of this timeline. The popular diagnosis in the 1980s was "Chronic Fatigue Syndrome." I bet you forgot about that one. When was the last time you heard of someone having it? Not recently, eh. Where did it go? What was the cure? In the 1990's ADD and ADHD came into full bloom, even though we were talking about it in the '80s. They've hung on pretty well too. But in the 2000's we began to see a lot of children with Bipolar Disorder.

We all function within a range on a scale. Atypical Asperger's is simply on a different part of that scale than most people are accustomed.

Here are some basic considerations if you question whether your child may have a form of Asperger's Syndrome:

Your child is bright but doesn't interact well with peers.

Your child doesn't have a normal filter when expressing himself. He says inappropriate things at inappropriate times.

He doesn't seem too bothered to be on the "outside" of things socially.

He is preoccupied or his focus on certain activities is abnormal or unusually intense.

He is preoccupied with parts of objects in a way that others are not.

His conversation runs to things that are completely dis-interesting to others, and he fails to notice.

This is not an exhaustive or comprehensive list. But it's a good start. Get a comprehensive assessment if you think this may be a problem.

SIGNS AND SYMPTOMS OF ASPERGER'S

Asperger's syndrome is considered as one of the pervasive developmental disorders and with the main signs and symptoms of Asperger's centering on the impairment of social and communicative abilities. Current statistics suggest that up to 3 out of every 10,000 children will be diagnosed with Asperger's syndrome and boys are 3 or 4 times more likely to suffer from the disorder than girls.

Here is a list of the most common signs and symptoms associated with Asperger's syndrome, but please bear in mind that every child's case of Asperger's is different and just because a majority of kids showed one symptom, doesn't mean every child has or will.

1. As stated above, a majority, but not all, of Asperger's syndrome symptoms, are social in nature. The first symptom that many parents or teachers notice in a child that has Asperger's is a lack of understanding of social cues or the inability to understand body language. This can extend to the basic ability to start and end a conversation as well as the idea of waiting to speak until the person you are speaking to has finished.

2. Most children that show signs of Asperger's syndrome do not like any change in their routine. This is also a common symptom of the classic form of autism, as well.

3. A common symptom that is almost always associated with Asperger's syndrome is the apparent lack of empathy. Empathy, or the ability to sense the emotions and emotional state of another person, is part of an Asperger's patient social failings. It is easy to see how a lack

of empathy can make even the simplest social interaction extremely awkward.

4. An Asperger's child may not be able to understand the subtle differences in tone and meaning during social interaction. It makes things like understanding humor or plays-on-words like puns almost impossible to understand. Also, things like sarcasm tend to be extremely difficult for an Asperger's child to understand.

The child may also not use the proper speech patterns and not vary their tone of speech much or at all. Again, this only adds to the social awkwardness of a child with this disorder.

5. Adding to the already overwhelming social awkwardness is the fact that many Asperger's sufferers will tend to use much more formal or advanced language for their age. While it might seem cute and even endearing when conversing with adults, with other children it can be extremely alienating.

6. A child with Asperger's syndrome also tends to avoid eye contact when speaking to you. They either look at the ground or

just look away from the person to whom they are speaking.

7. Despite these socially awkward traits, many Asperger's children will be quite talkative, usually about one topic that they may seem to be obsessed with. It can be something as simple as baseball stats or something obscure that they just saw on television.

8. They may also have an unusual posture or walking style and move in a clumsy manner.

While Asperger's syndrome doesn't present the serious problems that classic autism does, it can still be a very tough disorder to deal with. With the proper assistance, however, a child diagnosed with Asperger's can live a happy and full life.

Chapter 5: Ways That Adults Can Help A Child With As Understand What Is Said To Them

A child will find processing information a difficult thing to do. This is because they may find it difficult to understand the world around them. Even when the child with an AS does understand a situation, they may not understand the words that go with that situation. Sometimes it is easy to assume that the child understands what is being said to them because they appear to follow instructions. However, the likelihood is that the child will know what to do when instructions are given in certain contexts because they have done it numerous times previously.

There are several ways in which to enhance a child's comprehension of what people are saying to them.

Say less and say it slowly

The adult can limit the amount of works they use to communicate with the child but still communicate the relevant information. Use key works that are specific to the context of the situation, repeat and stress them and use gestures, such as pointing, to accompany them.

If the child has only recently begun to use speech as a means of communication, the adult should use single words to communicate with them. When using this method of communication it is important to label things when they are immediately given to the child. If the child's attention has shifted onto something else, the word will lose its meaning.

Using gestures to accompany language can also encourage the child to understand what is being said to them. For example, when offering the child a drink the adult should gesture the action of drinking by pretending to hold a glass in one hand and bringing it in their mouth as if they were taking a sip. A similar thing can be used for eating. Over exaggerated facial expressions can also be used along with shaking the head for "yes" and "no" and a waving of the hand for "hello" and "goodbye". When talking to the child about people, for example "grandma is staying"; it helps to present the child with a photo of who is being spoken about.

Other visual methods that can be used to increase understanding include picture timetables, line drawings, cue cards and object/picture schedules.

Using Augmentative and Alternative Communication (AAC) supports

AAC describes any form of language other than speech that assists a child in social communicative interactions. There is a large range of AAC devices available for children who have no speech, and these children themselves are very diverse. Therefore, it is essential that a team of appropriate individuals evaluate different AAC options with parents of a child with AS, before a decision about their use is made. Criteria that need to be discussed before an AAC device is implemented include, cognitive and motor abilities, learning style, communication needs and literacy ability.

Different types of AAC devices that are suitable for the child with ASD include:

Sign Language: There are several difference sign language systems, for example, American Sign Language (ASL), British Sign Language (BSL), MakatonTM, Paget Gorman Signed SpeechTM, and Signed Exact English. When using sign language with a child, it can be beneficial to use a total communication approach. Total communication is the use of combined speech and sign so that the same language structure is modeled for the child in two modalities. The use of total communication helps to highlight key word meanings and help language comprehension.

Interactive Communication Boards: They contain visual symbols organized by topic. They can be created in different sizes and formats depending on the activity and environment that they are needed for. They can be both portable and stationary; one board is designed to stay in one location. The selection and organization of the symbols that are used need to be motivating and chosen to enhance functional communication for the child.

Communication Cue Cards: Are primarily used with verbal children. They are used to remind the child what to say and to provide them with an alternative means to communication. They can contain one or more messages in pictorial or written form and can replace verbal prompts. They are therefore, particularly useful for children who are reliant on verbal prompts. Cue cards can work well in situations where the child with an ASD needs to express a message in a stressful situation.

Conversation Books: Can be pictorial or can consist of a written summary of conversation topics used for increasing conversational abilities. The conversational topics are organized in a small book, wallet or something similar and are used as a focus of conversation with an adult. It is important that the book is age appropriate and the topics chosen are meaningful to the child. This can often be achieved best using photographs, especially for the younger child. Conversation books work by organizing the conversation for the child. They provide a concrete, visual means to share and maintain topics.

Voice Output Communication Aids: Speech output devices give non-verbal children a 'voice'. A team of relevant professionals should determine the most appropriate technology option. Once this has been established, the team then needs to decide on an appropriate vocabulary selection, the layout of the device, the size of the symbols and the principal situation to encourage the child to use the device.

The combined use AAC, social supports, organizational supports and visually cued instruction can enhance the social communicative interactions in children.

: Coping with People with Asperger's

To get along with someone who has Asperger's, look closely at that annoying car.

You know when you are on the highway and everybody moves along like a ballet, merging, exiting, and changing lanes. There is moving over for a truck. There is moving away if you are blocking someone who wants to go faster than you. There are all kinds of unwritten rules we adhere to in order to not run each other over.

The Asperger car is the one on cruise control at exactly the speed limit. Technically, that is what everyone is supposed to do, but there are a million scenarios where if you refuse to slow down or speed up, you actually make everyone else's life hell.

But there is no way to tell that annoying car, "Hey, you're breaking the law," (because they're not) and you can't tell them, "Hey, you're being inconsiderate," (because they'll say, "Well, that merging car could have slowed down until I got by,"). You can't tell that car, "Hey, there are some unwritten rules you're not paying attention to." (They'll say like what? And then they will argue.)

So there's no way to tell the annoying car they're annoying because they actually don't understand the concept of annoying. They only understand the concept of right and wrong. People with Asperger's have an intense need to do the right thing the right way. But often they fail to see what that is.

People with Asperger's don't have friends
Someone with Asperger's doesn't feel a huge need to connect on an emotional level with lots of different people. They might think they are connecting emotionally. But it is not how other people do it.

Like, the Asperger father who never called to say he loves you, or the Asperger girlfriend who disappears for five days because she did not know you would expect her to be there. It's a friend who never calls or emails because they don't see communication as part of a friendship.

There are a million different ways people with Asperger's inadvertently isolate themselves from the world of friendship, but suffice it to say that while people with Asperger's have lots of depression and lots of anxiety, you'll rarely hear them say they need more friends.

It's overwhelming to be close to people. A lot of people with Asperger's who are married sleep in separate beds or have sex with minimal physical contact but you need to find the thing that's going to work for so you can have that one intimate relationship. Otherwise, you'll get older and realize everyone is paired off and there's no room for you to have your best friend because adult life best friends are spouses.

Tips for Loving Someone with Asperger's Syndrome

All romantic relationships have challenges and require some work. Being in a relationship with someone who has Asperger's syndrome can create an additional challenge. This is because the partners think and feel differently, leaving a lot of room for misunderstanding and miscommunication.

Here are three ideas you might find helpful: -

Don't put the blame on your partner: Your partner isn't solely to blame for your relationship problems. The true problems lie in the blending of two different modes of being.

Learn as much as you can about AS: If you don't know much about AS, it's easy to misinterpret your partner's actions and think they don't care about you. Educating yourself on how AS functions can be a huge help in better understanding your partner and feeling compassion toward them.

Reframe your partner's behavior: You might think that your partners know precisely what you need but purposely ignores it or intentionally does something to hurt you. And when you think your partner is cold and mean, you not only get upset and angry, but you also might view all of their actions and intentions negatively. Refraining from your partner'sbehavior helps you refocus on your relationship and work to improve it (vs. stewing in the negativity).

Chapter 6: The Impact Of Asperger's Syndrome Across The Lifespan

Asperger's Syndrome is both a developmental and behavioral disorder but not a mental disorder. A person diagnosed with this condition has the ability to function like everyone else but with certain impairments especially when it comes to relating with other people. For instance, he or she may have difficulties with making friends, establishing a connection with another person, following certain norms or social rules, as well as showing courtesy or respect in some contexts.

They also struggle with making sense of how someone should interact with another person. They find it difficult to effectively communicate both verbally and non-verbally. When you know someone that falls under the spectrum of Autism, you'll notice that in certain situations, their posture, body language, gestures, eye contact, or facial expressions might be a little "off",

The most ideal way to understand and cope with Asperger's is to find out how it affects a person throughout the different phases of life. The symptoms of Asperger's that become apparent differ across childhood, adolescence, and adulthood. Although the emergence of the symptoms varies depending on which developmental stage a person is in, people diagnosed with Asperger's generally struggle with dealing and relating with other people. This chapter is focused on enumerating the struggles or experiences that a child, teen and adult diagnosed with Asperger's go through.

Childhood

Problems with Communication

Children with Asperger's Syndrome look like much the other kids their age. They too can understand, comprehend and learn certain concepts at home and at school. However, because of their condition, they usually find it hard to communicate with others. They also struggle with behaving appropriately in certain situations. For example, kids with Asperger's can hear what other people are saying. They could also understand the meaning of the words that they are hearing. The reason why they are still considered socially awkward is because they cannot pick up non-verbal cues. This causes them to not get or understand the complete idea or message.

Social Skills need Improvement

Children with Asperger's are usually assumed by many as loners or introverts. However, this is not always the case. There are children with this condition who want to mingle and make friends but have problems with initiating contact. This often causes them to feel lonely and isolated. Also, other kids with this condition might not prefer playing with other children because they sometimes find it challenging and confusing. They may also prefer doing activities alone because it requires a minimal amount of social interaction. For instance, they might prefer playing video games, or using the computer rather than playing group sports or other recreational activities. Children with Asperger's also have the tendency to misunderstand a lot of social cues; a smile from their classmate might cause them to assume that the sender of the smile wants to be their best friend. When the sender plays with other kids, they might feel abandoned or disappointed because that person is playing with someone else.

It is a known fact that bullying has long been a problem in our society. However, a child with Asperger's Syndrome is at greater risk of being bullied. This is because they may not be able to communicate or express themselves properly. They are more prone to being picked on by other people because of their inability to recognize facial expressions or body language and determine whether a person is plotting to harm them or not. The bottom line is that children with Asperger's Syndrome need a lot of support and guidance when it comes to interacting with other people.

Typical Behavior

Keep in mind that children with Asperger's are just like other kids; they're still growing and just starting the process of discovering their interests, hobbies and passion. If you know a child with this condition, keep in mind that having a fixation on an object or an activity is a typical behavior of people with Asperger's Syndrome.

They may also be sensitive to noise, strong odor, or other things because they may sense things a little bit differently when compared with other people. They may also have difficulties with adapting to changes. They might be upset if their things are rearranged or if certain changes are made. They usually find it hard to adapt to sudden changes. They might also react violently or aggressively when things do not go exactly the way they expected them to be. If you know someone who is diagnosed with Asperger's you always have to have a lot of patience and understanding.

Compared with other kids that fall on the Autism Spectrum, children with Asperger's usually develop typically normal language and intellectual abilities. This is why some people deem Asperger's syndrome as the "hidden disorder". They even exert more effort with making friends and doing recreational activities with other people.

Adolescence

Individuals at an early adulthood stage tend to explore personal relationships. During early adulthood or college years, a person diagnosed with Asperger's Syndrome may live at home to prevent sudden changes in environment. They may join an interest-based group and gain communication skills through this avenue. They may choose a career that catches their interest and try to be in a single room at home to decrease too much social demands and also to aid in relaxation. There are a lot of developmental changes that are happening during this age and support groups should always be there to guide and help them.

College

Not all students may understand what this person is experiencing and not all will be patient. Therefore, the right college course is one big factor for the person with Asperger's Syndrome to excel and show his or her potential. It is essential that they are the ones who would decide the degree that they want to study in college. For instance, if they love solving mathematical equations and have exceptional logical skills, they can take engineering as their major. The goal is to guide them in determining the appropriate course for them.

College can be somehow overwhelming to people with Asperger's especially when they are far away from home and living on their own. Most college freshmen with Asperger's usually require the most amount of social support during their first years in the university. They may also want to join organizations or participate in social events but have difficulties in finding the right one for them as well as being introduced.

Adulthood

Most symptoms of this condition persist through adulthood but when treated properly, they become stable and manageable. Usually, individuals with Asperger's learn how to cope with the condition better as they age. Unlike during their childhood or teenage years, they are now more familiar with their own set of strengths and weaknesses. They now know which skills to focus on.

Adults with Asperger's syndrome usually have unique living and employment arrangements. Since some may still struggle with living independently, they sometimes need support from their loved ones especially in the areas of their lives that need improvement.

Chapter 7: Helping Loved Ones Cope With Asperger's Syndrome

To tell or not to tell?

For family, friends or co-workers, how would you tell a person that they have Asperger's Syndrome? Are you the right person to tell someone of the condition? Yes, definitely. Imagine yourself in their situation. What if, you were the one with Asperger's Syndrome, and you have no idea what the condition is or how to cope with it? Through the years of living with your undiagnosed condition, you just accepted the fact that you seem a little bit awkward to other people and that they can do a lot of things that you find too challenging to achieve? Wouldn't you feel frustrated, confused and disappointed with yourself?

You may even have questions such as: "Why am I acting different than other people?" "Why am I not good with social interaction?," "I cannot understand people whenever they are using non-verbal communication." Questions like these might confuse and frustrate a person with this condition. It is quite unfair for them not to know. It is their right as a person and as a patient to be informed if their condition becomes detrimental to the quality of their life.

Directly informing a person that he is displaying a peculiar behavior quite similar to the symptoms of Asperger's syndrome will not only be beneficial for him, but also to the significant people around him. This is because their becoming aware of their challenging behaviors will allow them to control, manage, and minimize them. Being on top of their health status would enable them to lessen the negative effects that are brought by their condition.

Even if they are formally diagnosed with having Asperger's syndrome, you should never underestimate them. They may need guidance and support when it comes to dealing with other people, but they do have their own share of skills and talents. Learning and being more familiar with their condition would allow them to properly socialize with others and seek for support groups or networks. They are known for being intelligent and highly functional people and should be given to chance to understand what they are going through. Moreover, they may ultimately learn about therapies and strategies on how to minimize or relieve the symptoms brought about by Asperger's Syndrome.

Tips for Understanding and Helping a Loved One with Asperger's Syndrome

Never forget that they have unique needs

One of the best techniques to help a loved one cope with his condition is to always remind yourself that they have certain limitations and needs that need to be addressed. For instance, they have a certain fondness for developing a routine. Since they find it difficult to understand, make sense or predict certain events or situations, having a routine gives them a little control over the conditions as well as an idea of the things that are yet to come. They often find changes or disruptions in their routine annoying and even frustrating. This is the main reason why parents or other primary caregivers need to gradually help the patient learn to adapt to change.

Remember that they process information differently

The brain of a normal person is capable of filtering the massive amount of information it receives. It is able to determine which information needs to be processed and automatically disregards the ones that it finds irrelevant or insignificant. However, this is not the case for people with Asperger's. A lot of individuals with this condition struggle with sifting through relevant and irrelevant information. This is why you should be extra patient and understanding with them especially when you are teaching them new skills or concepts.

Work around their strengths

It is common knowledge that some people that are diagnosed with Asperger's are also considered as "savants". Savants are people with exceptional abilities. As a parent or guardian, you can contribute a lot to the development of their skills and abilities. One technique is to familiarize yourself with their strengths and interests. This would allow you to modify your teaching methods so that it would fit their learning style. They would also learn and understand things better when an approach is tailored to their unique needs and characteristics.

Allot time for yourself

Caring for another being involves a lot of struggles and difficulties. What more if he or she has special needs that require a lot more effort, patience and understanding? Looking after someone and attending to all his or her needs can sometimes be physically, mentally and emotionally draining. This is why it is important to still have some alone time. Planning a leisure hour or a relaxing day for yourself will enable you to feel renewed and empowered. Even if your child or loved one requires lot more of your support and guidance, you should still manage to look after your own health and needs.

Things to Remember:

☐ Once diagnosed, it is a must for the affected person to know all about the condition.

☐ Focus on their strengths and potentials to boost their self-confidence, but at the same time tell them their weaknesses so there can be a room for improvement.

☐ The earlier you reveal the real diagnosis to the person, the easier it is for him or her to accept things.

☐ We must put ourselves in their shoes for us to understand their condition. Empathy is a huge piece to offering support.

☐ We must remember that a person with Asperger's Syndrome should be treated with respect and patience.

☐ No one is perfect. So what we can do is to offer our helping hand, support them all the way and guide them until they learn how to cope with the pressure brought about by Asperger's Syndrome.

The more you know about Asperger's syndrome, the more you become capable of providing the love, support and guidance that they need.

Chapter 8: Misunderstandings And Misjudgments Of The Social Surroundings

In the previous chapters, we discussed how other people may perceive and understand their own interpersonal relationships with people suffering from Asperger Syndrome. It is now time to discuss and provide solutions to these various misunderstandings, misconceptions and misjudgments of society.

Tackling these issues in a chronological order, we need to begin with infancy and childhood. More advanced societies have no problem taking their children to a doctor for an examination if they suspect that there might be something wrong with their child. But less developed societies face a serious problem, that of social isolation.

The human species may have advanced away from the Spartan society (which murdered all the children that even looked like they were not strong enough to survive the Spartan lifestyle), but societies and religions still exist where any form of mental illness is treated with the incarceration to a lunatic asylum. Sufferers may be given some food and left there, unattended, until the end of his or her days.

Despite the efforts to educate and familiarize societies with the concept that not all mental disorders present a danger to society through violent and criminal behavior, there are still people that believe that any person suffering from such a disorder is a curse or an abomination and should be treated as such. For various reasons (most of them pertaining to fear, lack of knowledge, religion and distrust of doctor's opinions) many societies choose not to accept aspies within their ranks.

Let us repeat and emphasize these facts about people suffering from Asperger Syndrome:
1) Most often, they are the victims of manipulation, bullying and extortion. This, by definition, means that under no circumstances do aspies present a danger to society and other people. They may present a danger to themselves, but that's as far as it goes!
2) In the vast majority of cases, they do not even appear in public unless they have to. And, again, in most of their social appearances, either they are not noticed, or if they do, it's just by speaking in a monotonous tone or clinging to a single topic. How can this be considered dangerous to society?
3) If we cannot accept that they suffer from a disorder and that it is not their fault that they do, we cannot be considered empathetic humans ourselves. We do to them exactly what we accuse them of doing to us: being insensitive and disregarding of the feelings of other people.

Unfortunately, no matter what is said, religious fanaticism is a trait that will take a lot more than communication about medical conditions to change, and it is really a matter of serious debate why people do not trust doctors. To conclude on this point, people should not fear or be ashamed to take their children for an examination if they suspect that there might be something wrong. One of the most important aspects of proper treatment of the syndrome is that the correct diagnosis is made as early as possible.

And now we need to address another important and related issue, pride and scandal. It's time to discuss those parents who consider it a blow to their own pride that their children display the symptoms of Asperger's and those parents that think that if the world learns about their child's condition, it will create a scandal.

Parents are supposed to love their children no matter what. And they are expected to do everything to ensure their welfare and wellbeing. They must also do everything in their power to see to it that any medical problems that may appear during childhood are dealt with.

Many parents have been heard saying, or rather, shouting, "This child cannot be mine!" Why? Because he or she displays symptoms of a syndrome for which they are not even responsible? Because it might be the parents themselves that transferred the genetic heritage to their offspring? Because it was just bad luck that this condition happened?

No matter what the responses to these questions might be, it happened. Now what? Just leave them be? Lock them up some place that no one will ever learn of their existence? Is that human behavior? Is that human decency? And we use the term human and not parental. No matter what happened, parents must be parents, and do whatever it takes for their children to thrive.

They cannot let their pride or the fear of a scandal interfere with the timely diagnosis of the problem and the intervention that may be the key to a normal life for the child. It's not a matter of name, money and history; it's a matter of human dignity.

The second point to be made is school. Sometimes, aspies are more advanced than the rest of the children at school in the fields of mathematics, chemistry, biology or other classes. There have been many cases which document that people suffering from mental disorders are extremely adept and notice things that others miss.

For them, the subject matter which is taught in the classroom may be mundane and boring. Typical homework assignments may even be frustrating. This does not mean that the students are arrogant, spiteful or insubordinate, as some teachers consider them to be and punish them accordingly. It only means that some other method must be devised to maintain their interest in the field and help them advance further.

Punishment and chastising can only result in negative situations for aspies, and this may make some perfectly good individuals with great prospects withdraw and isolate themselves from society and never accomplish anything. If teachers cannot understand by themselves or be taught in seminars how they should handle aspies, then special schools may be in order. It is question worthy what would happen to Nobel Prize winner Vernon L. Smith, if his teachers did not recognize his potential for accomplishment.

It is even more worrisome how many other Vernon L. Smiths disappeared because their teachers, and the reactions they received at school in general, forced them to withdraw to solitude.

The biggest shortcoming is the lack of support and understanding for these people. They are not evil, they are not dangerous and they are not devils. They are just people suffering from a disorder that they did not cause themselves.

Most of the problems and the symptoms pertaining to the patients of the Asperger Syndrome are limited to childhood and adolescence in more than 50% of cases. After adulthood, the problems may lessen or even disappear. Adult aspies actually have decided for themselves to do something about how society perceives them.

Some people view their opinions as extreme. Some others agree with them. Most others are indifferent. These opinions are presented in internet sites like **Wrong Planet**, while a subculture of aspies has been formed to allow them to communicate and exchange their views freely.

The main claim that aspies bring forth is that they should be recognized as different and not as people suffering from a disorder or a disability. For them, Asperger Syndrome is similar to homosexuality and people that display the symptoms should be treated and respected likewise. They claim that just like homosexuality was removed from the standard Diagnostic and Statistical Manual, so should Asperger's be removed.

To their cause, they have enlisted some very prominent figures, like that of the University of Cambridge Professor of Developmental Psychopathology **Simon**

Baron-Cohen, who is also a Fellow of Trinity College. His view on the subject as published in a paper in 2002, is:

"In society, there may be no great benefit by an eye with an ability for precise detail. But in mathematics, cataloging, music, computing, engineering and science in general, and eye for detail would probably lead to success, greatness and accomplishment rather than failure."

According to Baron-Cohen, there are only two reasons to keep the classification of aspies as a disorder or a disability. The first one is to maintain the provisions for the special support that is legally required, and the second is to recognize the emotional difficulties that result from the reduced empathy exhibited by aspies.

He concludes his views by mentioning that the genes behind Asperger's combination of abilities have existed throughout the human history and that they have made remarkable contributions to its evolution.

The concept behind the whole debate is that there neither is, nor ever should be, a brain configuration that is considered to be "ideal" and that normal people should comply with. Nor should any deviation from what is considered normal by considered as a pathology to be treated and remedied.

Just like the term "**neurotypical**" is used to describe people with normal neurological development, the term "**neurodiverse**" should be used to describe people with neurological developments that are considered to be deviating from the normal parameters.

It seems that there is a marked difference between adult aspies, who seem not to want to be changed and are actually proud of their diversity, and the parents who consider

Asperger Syndrome a problematic situation that needs to be resolved at all costs (assuming that there are no pride and scandal issues involved).

No matter what the outcome of this debate might be at the level of legislature and regulation, the basis of the issue should be that it is neither a shame nor a curse if a child suffers from AS. At least this is what **Liane Holiday Willey** maintains in her books on the subject.

This is a story worth looking at. Liane Willey was born in 1959. She went through life and nobody noticed her abnormalities for forty years! She was diagnosed with Asperger's in 1999. And what did she do about it? She published:

"Pretending to be Normal" **in 1999**

"Asperger Syndrome in the Family: Redefining Normal" **in 2001**

"Adolescents and Asperger Syndrome in the Adolescent Years: Living with the Ups and Downs and Things in Between" **in 2003**

"Safety Skills for Asperger Women: How to Save a Perfectly Good Female Life" **in 2011**

She also founded the Asperger Society of Michigan.

If Willey fits the definition of evil, the devil or a danger, then these terms must be redefined and radically at that. However, it would probably be a lot easier to separate Siamese children than try to change centuries' long religious indoctrination and dogmatic view on what is or what is not normal.

Another despairing fact was shown in a study conducted in England in 2007. The general population may be aware of what autism and Asperger Syndrome are, but they have never been informed or educated about the experience of actually living with one. Similar studies were conducted in other countries with likewise results.

These studies indicate that there is a serious lack of publications which would inform the public of what needs to be done when they are faced with a situation where they must interact with an aspie. The vast majority of the available published works deal with the definitions and the nuances **but not usable advice or information about actions**.

These studies go one step further in mentioning that the general population has only been advised about autism and the autism spectrum and that very few people are actually aware that there is a marked difference between general autism and Asperger Syndrome. In fact, most people have not even heard the term.

What is even more frustrating for the aspies and their families is the conclusion of thesis studies. The vast majority of the general population responded, to the relevant questions, that they would be far more in favor and accepting of a person displaying the Asperger symptoms if they had previously been informed about it. If they were taught what they were supposed to do and how they would need to address aspies, they would be more comfortable and willing to modify their behaviors.

It is obvious that a systematic effort must be devised to educate the general population about Asperger's syndrome (and autism in general), not only as a condition or a disability but also as a form of living that requires some attention and some effort from those that society calls normal and science calls "neurotypical."

If this gets under way, the next time a person meets someone who speaks in a monotonous voice about a single topic and seems to not pay attention to attempts to change the topic, he or she may understand that they are not dealing with a person with a weird personality trait but an individual who may be suffering from the symptoms of Asperger's. And they may choose to adjust their behavior accordingly, instead of getting incensed.

Therapies and Medication

For the time being and until the issues that we discussed in the previous chapters are resolved, Asperger Syndrome is considered as a disorder, and it's being managed by mainstream medicine through therapies and medication. The focus of the various treatments is to reduce the symptoms and to teach age-appropriate skills which may be missing from the patient.

As aforementioned, the therapies that may be used involve a multidisciplinary set of therapists and doctors in treatments that are prescribed on a case-by-case basis, as there is no single course of action which would cover the syndrome in general. Unfortunately, the data pertaining to how much progress has or has not been made is limited and it's inadvisable to extract any conclusions.

Medication

The nature of the syndrome, and the symptoms exhibited and pertaining to Asperger's itself, are not treatable by any medication. What needs medication and is treated accordingly is the existence of any comorbid conditions that, if left untreated, will result in more serious problems. This is but one more reason it is most imperative to diagnose the correct conditions as early as possible and why it is necessary for more than one doctor to get involved in the diagnostic process.

In many cases, the syndrome is accompanied with anxiety, depression, inattention and aggression. For these cases the atypical antipsychotics **risperidone** and **olanzapine** have displayed effectiveness in reducing the associated symptoms. Risperidone reduces the repetitive behavior which can induce self-injuries, can limit the outbursts of aggression and impulsiveness, and improve behaviors in social relationships and stereotypical patterns.

To improve on the restrictive and repetitive interests and behaviors, selective serotonin reuptake inhibitors (SSRIs) such as **fluvoxamine, fluoxetine** and **sertraline** have also proved effective.

There is one more issue to discuss in reference to medications. The occurrence of side effects is, in many cases, difficult to evaluate and may be dangerous. Patients of the autism spectrum are also routinely excluded from the tests and evaluations of the effectiveness of these medications against comorbid conditions.

Such side effects include an abnormal metabolism, an increased risk of type 2 diabetes, serious long-term neurological conditions and problems in cardiac conduction times. SSRIs may also have the opposite effect than the desired outcome regarding impulsiveness, aggression and sleep problems. Taking risperidone may result in weight gain and fatigue, which increase the risk of restlessness and dystonia. The use of sedatives may also have an impact in the learning process at school.

As amply displayed, medication, unless there are other conditions present, can be used only on certain occasions and to treat very specific situations. Otherwise, they may cause more problems than those they are called upon to solve. Treatment of AS relies heavily on the implementation of other cognitive therapies.

Therapies

For a total treatment of AS, many different therapies must be coordinated and focused together on addressing the core symptoms, such as the poor communication skills and the restrictive and repetitive routines. Linguistic capabilities, verbal strengths and deficiencies, and nonverbal inadequacies must also be taken under serious consideration.

The typical treatment program includes:

1) Applied Behavioral Analysis

ABA (previously known as **behavioral modification**) is a set of techniques implemented to systematically intervene and modify abnormal social behaviors. In the case of AS, the technique used is intended as **social skills training** and its purpose is to improve interpersonal interactions and any other skills pertaining to or interfering with communication between people.

The main concept behind the application of ABA to people with Asperger's is the hypothesis that there is absence of a **theory of mind.** In abbreviation, TOM. is the ability to understand that a person's brain works in a series of mental states such as beliefs, intents, desires, knowledge, pretensions, etc., and that other persons operate in the same mental states as well. These conditions of the mind are different from person to person and the focus of the therapy is to make one person understand and accept his or her own mental states as well as those of others.

In this regard, children displaying Asperger's are a bit luckier than children displaying the symptoms of the other disorders of the autism spectrum, as their initial understanding of a social theory of mind is considerably higher.

The therapy focuses on theory of mind tasks. The concept is that the abilities involved in mental processes are subserved by a series of dedicated mechanisms. It is believed that these mechanisms are actually affected by the impairment, and not the cognitive functions themselves.

By assigning the TOM tasks, the hypothesis is that these dedicated mechanisms, which may otherwise be inactive, are put to work and serve their purposes, which is to support the overlaying cognitive functions. Consequently, the cognitive functions allow the individual to first comprehend about his or her own states of mind and then to understand how these mental states translate from one person to another.

2) Cognitive Behavioral Therapy

This is a common therapeutic tactic in all disorders that have to do with the brain.

The objective is to improve **stress management** in reference to anxiety, depression and the emotions that produce explosive outbursts. The intervention also aims to reduce the obsessive occupation with interests and the constant repetition of the daily routines.

The objective of CBT is to improve everyday functioning. To achieve that goal it uses a number of techniques and physiotherapies. These fall under two major models.

The transactional model considers the stress as an imbalance between the demands made to one person and the resources this person has at his disposal to satisfy the demands. The problem occurs when the applied pressure on a person exceeds his or her ability to cope with the situation. The model focuses on this ability to cope with the problem and intervenes so that the stressing factor can be considered as a positive or even challenging notion instead of a threat.

The health realization (or innate health) model focuses on the thought processes, which determine the appropriate response to what is perceived as a potentially stressful situation.

In both models, there are over thirty techniques available, oriented to allow the person undergoing therapy to better manage his or her stress. A brief list of the techniques which are most used in AS therapies, looks like:

Autogenic training
Conflict resolution
Cranial release
Social activity
Mindfulness
Nootropics
Artistic expression
Somatics training
Time management
Planning and decision making
Pets

3) Occupational or Physical Therapy

If any person anywhere and at any time finds any doctor of any discipline that will ever say that physical exercise is not a good thing, it should be a surprise of great magnitude. In the case of AS, these therapies aim at improving the sensory perception and the motor coordination abilities that are woefully absent, and are important in improving the psychological conditions rather than the physical ones.

One of the symptoms exhibited by aspies is physical clumsiness. **Sensory processing** is the sequence of events in the neurological system that interprets the input from the environment through the sensors of the body, and allows it to be used and interpreted in the most effective way.

The therapy intends to teach an aspie how to use his or her brain to process the modality input from multiple sources and understand concepts like:

a)
Proprioception
This is the understanding of the relative position of the various parts of the body and the amount of effort required for movement.

b) Tactile
This is the understanding of the various sensations and emotions caused by the

touch of the human body receptors to thermal, chemical, mechanical and light sources.

c) Olfactory

Similar to tactile, this has to do with the input provided by various odors and smells.

d) Vestibular system

This is the system in the body that is responsible for balance and spatial orientation. (Remember that aspies may not be able to walk in a tandem gait.)

e)

Interoception

This is the normal and physiological capacity of any living organism to receive information and convert them to perception and then action or reaction and, consequently, be able to convert them to usable functions.

Motor coordination is the physical process that allows the human body to receive the inputs from kinematic and kinetic parameters and to form an intended action. A kinematic parameter references the spatial direction and a kinetic parameter references the amount of force required to move towards a certain point. A similar combination of parameters is the visual input from a moving object and the range of motion to be carried by the hand, which will allow it to capture the object that the eye is watching.

To put it simply, motor coordination is the process that allows the mind to order the body to make a motion, based on the input it receives through the five senses.

Aspies have problems in the neural process of the cerebellum which do not allow them to interpret the sensory input and, therefore, to order the body to take action. The therapy focuses on instructing the brain how to correctly perceive the input and then how to react accordingly.

4) Speech Therapy

We have repeatedly mentioned the way aspies speak. Specialized speech therapy is aimed at acquainting the aspie with the pragmatics of give-and-take during a normal conversation so that they no longer disregard or misinterpret the stance of the person to whom they are talking.

The therapy is to be administered by a speech-language pathologist. While the therapy should primarily focus on the pragmatics, lesser issues may involve therapy in:

1) Phonation

This is the sound production in the larynx. We have already discussed that when aspies talk, their voice may sound in a way that alienates the listener.

2) Resonance

The pitch of a voice is a matter of resonance. Aspies may talk without pitch. This part is aimed to introduce the importance of pitch in a voice pattern.

3) Fluency

When an aspie talks, he may sound incoherent. This part of the therapy is intended to match words with meanings.

4) Intonation

The monotonous style of speech is addressed in this part of the therapy.

5) Pitch variance

Pitch is an emotion indicator. Each pitch is associated with a different emotion.

6) Morphology

This is the part of the therapy which teaches how to speak in small sentences which make sense, using grammar and syntax rules.

To return to the pragmatics aspect of the therapy, this is the central part, as it teaches the ways by which context is transformed to meaning. Remember that sometimes, people suffering from the syndrome do not understand the meanings of what they are actually saying. Also, they do not have a grasp of sarcastic speech, metaphors, humor and other forms of conversational implicature.

These pragmatics are actually what teaches all people to speak in a way so that others can understand what they are saying and react to it.

5) Positive behavior support

This part of the therapy is not aimed at the patient. It is aimed at the families and the faculties at school, and its objective is to introduce behavioral management strategies to be used at home or school to support and tolerate the behavioral problems of an aspie.

The basic notion behind the training is to understand what lies behind and maintains the abnormal behavior. These behaviors serve a purpose for the aspies; they are functional. Children do not have to be suffering from the syndrome to display a certain behavior in the presence of adults in order to receive more attention and/or rewards.

The key is functional behavior assessment. It describes behaviors, marks the context in reference to time, events and circumstances, and predicts when the abnormal behavior will occur or not. The training involves:

1) Identification of Goals

This is a two-prong effort. The first leg is to identify if the strategy selected is feasible in reference to the individual it will be implemented with, desirable by the individual (it will do no good if the patient resents it), and effective in obtaining the second leg, which is the specific behavioral adjustments that are needed.

2) Gathering of Information

An integral part of the effectiveness of any strategy is the correct observation of the behaviors at home and at school in association with the context issues. Behavioral patterns in aspies are repetitive, which means that there may be a certain time during the day that the abnormal behavior occurs. Or, a child displaying the symptoms may be perfectly normal until a derogatory comment or a bad joke is made, and then he or she becomes insulted and acts without thinking. Additionally, a class in school may be considered too mundane and boring for an aspie, and a different set of curricular activities may have to be devised to match his skills in a specific field.

All the above is necessary information so that the model of positive behavioral support implemented will produce the optimal effect.

3) Development of a Working Hypothesis

The first two of these steps yield the appropriate information, which, under examination by an appropriate team of professionals, will determine the specific issues pertaining to the individual aspie who will undergo these strategic changes. There is a marked difference in the underlying dysfunctionality between an aspie who is focused and orderly and an aspie who cannot focus on anything and is completely disorderly.

4) Designing a Support Plan

After all the above steps have been completed, it is time to decide on what to do. How can a behavior occurring only at a specific time of the day be handled in a focused and orderly child? How can he or she handle a bad joke or a derogatory comment when he or she is completely impulsive?

This, and the implementation step, are actually the most important ones in the positive support training. If the wrong plan is devised, then no matter how well it is implemented, it is the wrong plan. It will yield no positive results.

5) Implementation

Once parents and teachers know what to do, they need to actually do it. They need to do it properly and most of all **willingly**. An aspie will sense if the instructions and the behavior of the parent or the teacher is forced, or resentful, or performed without their hearts in it. They will disregard the strategy altogether.

Assuming that the correct plan has been devised, both parents and teachers must, first of all, be convinced that it will provide the desired results. Then they must project the feeling that they will do whatever it takes gladly and wholeheartedly.

The implementation involves one last element which is the trickiest of them all: patience. If parents and teachers expect results immediately, they will be completely and utterly disappointed. Part of the training is to make them understand that it will not only take time to see improvements, but it may also be that despite their efforts, their child may show very little to no improvement at all, if the case is severe enough.

This part is especially tricky because many people are inherently impatient. They must first achieve this virtue themselves before being allowed to implement any strategy for positive behavior support on another individual.

6) Monitoring

The last issue of the training is to monitor the progress. This step will identify if the devised plan and its implementation were effective. If not, a revision may be required or the strategy may be altered altogether. Otherwise, just some tweaking may be required to some aspects of the strategy.

Therapies do not work on auto-pilot. There might be unintentional side-effects. These must be identified in the monitoring process and dealt with appropriately. And the most integral part of this process is that the parent and the teacher must always be in constant and immediate contact with the appropriate professionals who can guide and advise them in a proper and timely manner.

It is curious and noteworthy that the majority of the studies conducted on programs of early intervention that are behavior based are merely simple case reports of up to five participants. In most instances, they examine only a few problematic behaviors such as self-inflicted injuries, aggression, refusal to comply, spontaneous language and stereotypes, and completely ignore the existence of unintentional side-effects.

Other issues may have surfaced during the implementation of these therapies that were completely unexpected and, thus far, unexplained. For example, in a controlled study of the positive behavior support, a group of parents were trained in a one day workshop, while another group attended six individual lessons. The parents that attended the workshop reported **fewer** behavioral problems, while the parents that attended the individual lessons, reported **less intense** behavioral problems.

Such issues only reinforce the notion that there can be no single therapy for Asperger Syndrome, not only because aspies are very different from individual to individual, but also because those who are providing support, tolerance and understanding have a different level of comprehension of the nuances involved and a different attitude towards the implementation of the therapies.

As long as the core causes of the syndrome are not identified and medically or genetically dealt with, this will probably be the case, unless something really dramatic happens. Each individual case of a person that displays the symptoms of Asperger's will have to be treated differently and according to the specifics and the circumstances surrounding the specific individual.

Conclusion

I believe that you are now informed on how to handle a child or an adult with Asperger's syndrome.

Children who suffer from Asperger's syndrome take a lot of time to grow to maturity. You will therefore be patient with them as they grow. It is important for parents to know that and therefore the expectation for them to behave according to their age should not be there.

So it will be absurd to expect your child with this condition to behave their age. Before then, probably you found yourself between a rock and hard place on how to handle these cases. But I believe you a better placed to take care of this children or adults in giving them care after reading this book.

www.ingramcontent.com/pod-product-compliance
Lightning Source LLC
LaVergne TN
LVHW011950070526
838202LV00054B/4869